101 Glam Girl Ways to an Ultra Chic Lifestyle

WRITTEN BY
DAWN DEL RUSSO

ILLUSTRATED BY
BARBARA ANN SCARRILLO

Library of Congress Control Number:
2009908893

ISBN: 1-4392-5633-0

BookSurge Publishing
7290-B Investment Drive
N. Charleston, SC 29418

Illustrations by Barbara Ann Scarrillo

Book design by Armand P. Veneziano
APV Design Studio

Printed in the United States of America

To purchase additional copies of this book
please go to: www.belladawn.com
or contact BookSurge Publishing at
www.booksurge.com
or visit www.amazon.com

Acknowledgements

THIS BOOK IS DEDICATED TO MY SISTER, MY BEST FRIEND AND MY BEAUTY CONSULTANT, DENISE, THANK YOU FOR INSPIRING ME, KEEPING ME ON TRACK AND REMINDING ME YOU ONLY LIVE ONCE. LOVE YOU.

THANK YOU TO MY FATHER FOR TEACHING ME TO GO AFTER MY PASSION, MY MOM FOR BELIEVING IN MY DREAMS, AND JOE FOR TRUSTING IN ALL MY ENDEAVORS. MY FAMILY AND FRIENDS YOU ARE MY SUPPORT SYSTEM, THE DRIVING FORCE THAT CREATED THIS BEAUTIFUL REALITY CALLED LIFE.

THANK YOU SABRINA FOR THE OPPORTUNITY TO WORK TOGETHER AND CREATE THE BUZZ. RICH, THANK YOU FOR GUIDING ME ON THE PATH TO MANIFEST MY IMAGINATION. BARBARA ANN AND ARMAND, YOU MADE MY WORDS COME TO LIFE, I THANK YOU TRULY.

Introduction

Every Girl

WANTS TO LIVE A GLAMOROUS LIFESTYLE,
WHETHER IN THE LAP OF LUXURY OR ON A TIGHT BUDGET.

101 Glam Girl Ways to an Ultra Chic LifeStyle

PROVIDES QUICK, CHEEKY TIPS, TO LIVE THAT SWANK LIFESTYLE.
PUT TOGETHER SIMPLY,
EACH ONE-LINER TIP IS ILLUSTRATED
WITH CHARMING FASHIONABLE SKETCHES.
YOU WILL INDULGE IN THIS DELIGHTFUL QUICK READ!
IT IS JUST PERFECT FOR CONFIDENT WOMEN WITH A FLAIR
FOR FASHION AND DIVINE LIVING.

101 Glam Girl Ways to an Ultra Chic LifeStyle

IS EVERY WOMAN'S SECRET GUIDE
TO BREEZING THROUGH LIFE GLAMOROUSLY.
YOU WILL BE DELIGHTED WITH
COLORFUL ILLUSTRATIONS AND QUICK WITTY TIPS,

Its the Ultimate Secret Pocket Guide.

YOU CAN EASILY INCORPORATE THE TIPS INTO YOUR LIFE
TO MAKE IT A LITTLE SWEETER!

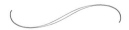

About the Illustrator

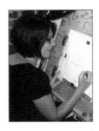

Barbara Ann Scarrillo

BARBARA ANN SCARRILLO HAS SPENT
OVER 20 YEARS DESIGNING
STYLISH LOGOS, AND ARTWORK IN THE
NEW YORK CITY AREA.
SHE GRADUATED FROM
THE FASHION INSTITUTE OF TECHNOLOGY
AND TURNED HER PASSION
INTO HER BUSINESS "BRUSHSTROKES".
BARBARA ANN'S WORDS TO LIVE BY:
" NEVER GET TOO BUSY MAKING A LIVING
THAT YOU FORGET TO MAKE A LIFE."

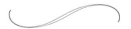

About the Author

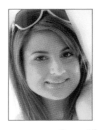

Dawn Del Russo

FASHION STYLIST DAWN DEL RUSSO,
OWNER OF BELLA DAWN BOUTIQUE,
AMBITIOUSLY TURNED HER CHILDHOOD
DREAM OF A "LUXE" BOUTIQUE INTO REALITY
AFTER COMPLETING HER B.S. IN BUSINESS MANAGEMENT.
DAWN HAS BEEN FEATURED IN NATIONAL PRINT MEDIA, INSTYLE, ELLE,
COSMO, US WEEKLY, AND LUCKY, AND NATIONAL TELEVISION FOX 5.
HER KNOWLEDGE AND STYLE ADVICE HAS SUCCESSFULLY LED HER TO
STYLE TRENDY, CHIC FASHIONS RECOGNIZED
INTERNATIONALLY AT WWW.BELLADAWN.COM.
SHE IS A CONTRIBUTING FASHION WRITER FOR SELECT ONLINE
MAGAZINES AS WELL AS HER OWN BLOG
WWW.MYINTIMATEAFFAIRWITHFASHION.COM.
SHE HAS A CHIC SENSE OF STYLE AND IS DEDICATED TO HELPING WOMEN
FIND THEIR INNER BEAUTY, CONFIDENCE, AND STYLE
STARTING FROM THE OUTSIDE APPEARANCE.
DAWN'S WORDS TO LIVE BY:
" TRUST IN YOUR DREAMS, BELIEVE IN YOUR PASSION,
AND THE WORLD IS YOURS."

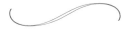

Tip#1

Wear Diamond Studs

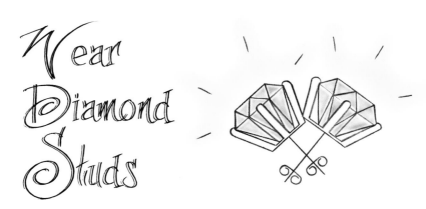

A LITTLE SPARKLE PEEKING THROUGH
WILL GRAB JUST THE RIGHT ATTENTION

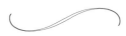

Flaunt Luscious Lashes

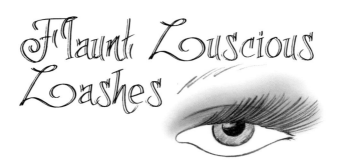

BEAUTIFUL LONG LASHES ARE A MUST
WEARING MASCARA OPENS UP YOUR EYES
AND DRAWS ATTENTION

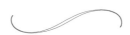

Wear What You Love

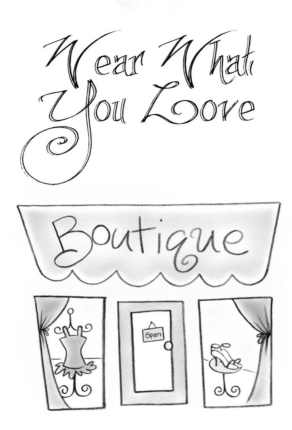

DON'T ALWAYS GO FOR DESIGNER NAMES
LOOK FOR SPLENDID PIECES IN UNDISCOVERED BOUTIQUES

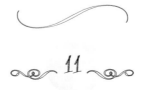

Tip #4

Mix It Up

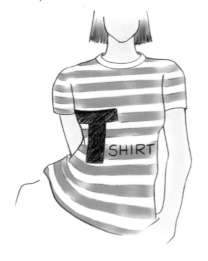

PAIR HIGH-END PIECES WITH LESS PRICEY ITEMS
NO ONE WILL SUSPECT YOUR OUTFIT
CAME FROM A BARGAIN STORE

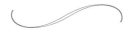

Change Up Your Hair Style

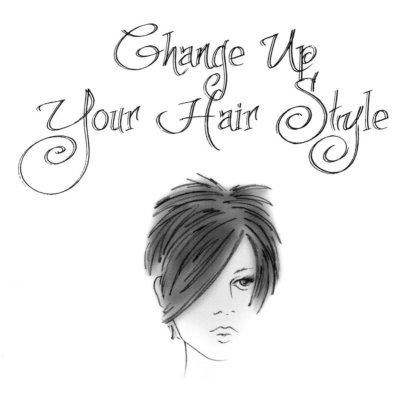

EVERY 6 WEEKS FRESHEN UP WITH A HAIR CUT
AND KEEP YOUR COLOR TOP NOTCH TOO

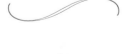

Tip#6

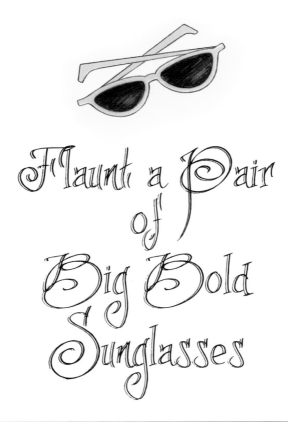

Flaunt a Pair of Big Bold Sunglasses

THEY HIDE A LATE NIGHT OUT AND LOOK ULTRA GLAM

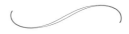

A Dust of Shimmer

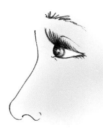

ADD A POP OF SHIMMER
IN KEY PLACES, LIKE
THE INNER CORNERS OF YOUR EYES
AND THE TOPS OF YOUR CHEEKBONES

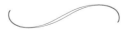

Tip#8

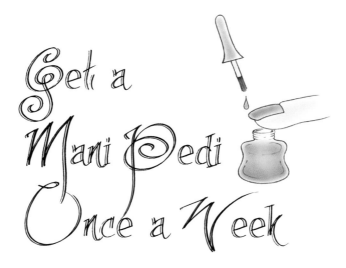

Get a Mani Pedi Once a Week

FOR THOSE NOT IN THE KNOW
A MANICURE/PEDICURE
IS A MAINTENANCE MUST

Buy the

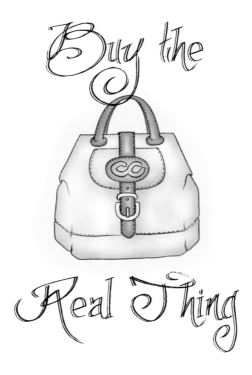

Real Thing

DON'T DO KNOCK OFFS
THEY ARE OH SO OBVIOUS AND TACKY

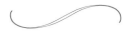

Always Wear Lip Gloss

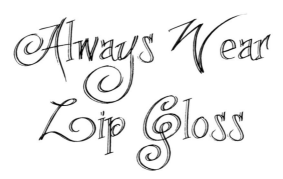

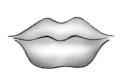

DRAW SOME ATTENTION TO YOUR SWEET POUT
PUCKER UP AND PUT SOME ON!

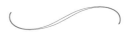

Tip #11

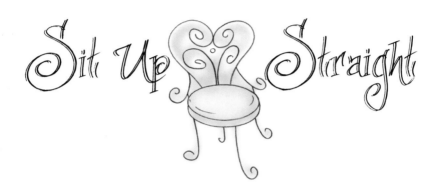

Sit Up Straight

GREAT POSTURE IS IMPORTANT
YOU WILL INSTANTLY LOOK FABULOUS

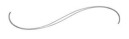

Tip#12

Wear a Classic White Button Down Blouse

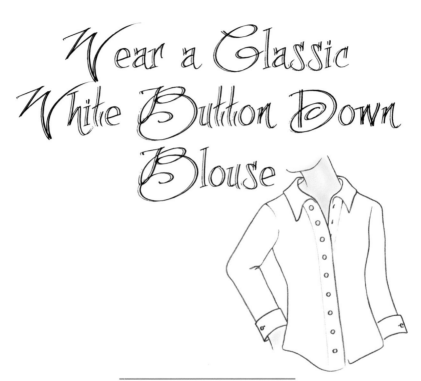

IT SHOULD BE A STAPLE
IN EVERY CLOSET FOR THE
"I HAVE NOTHING TO WEAR" DAY

Tip #13

The "Must Have" Little Black Dress

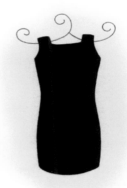

FIND ONE YOU LOVE AND HAVE IT TAILORED
TO FIT YOUR CURVES PERFECTLY

Learn a Second

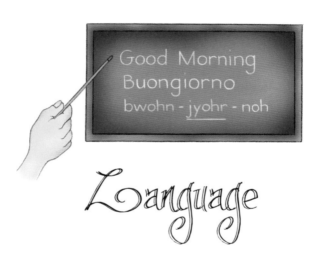

Language

FRENCH IS PREFERRED, BUT SPEAKING ANY LANGUAGE
FLUENTLY WILL UP YOUR CHIC FACTOR

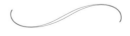

Tip #15

Wax Your Eyebrows

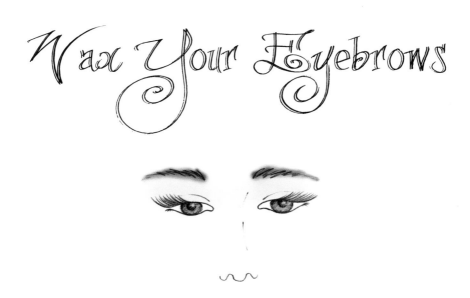

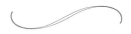

THIS IS NECESSARY MAINTENANCE
THAT WILL OPEN UP YOUR ENTIRE FACE

Tip #16

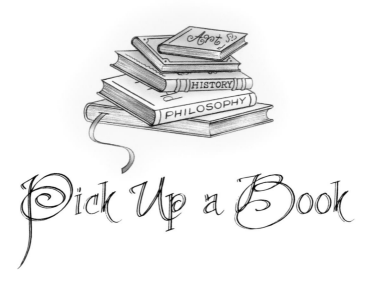

Pick Up a Book

KNOWLEDGE IS POWER
AND POWER IS CHIC

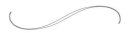

Tip#17

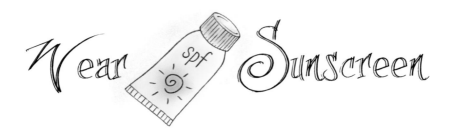

Wear Sunscreen

KEEP YOUR SKIN YOUNG, HEALTHY,
AND SUPPLE; WEAR SPF 15+.
MAKE THIS A DAILY REGIME

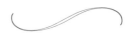

Tip#18

Brush Up 3x a Day

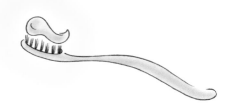

BRUSH YOUR TEETH WITH A WHITENING TOOTHPASTE
WHITE TEETH - YOUNGER LOOK

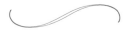

Carry a Small Clutch

THROW A SMALL CLUTCH IN YOUR LARGE BAG
FOR A QUICK CHANGE
FROM DAY TO EVENING.

Tip #20

Wear Sexy Lingerie

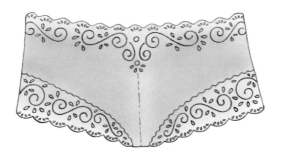

THEY MAKE YOU FEEL SO GOOD
AND ARE A TREAT FOR THAT SPECIAL SOMEONE

Tip#21

Use Hand

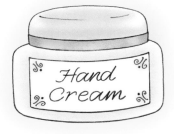

Cream

HANDS ARE THE MOST NOTICEABLE
SPOT FOR AGING; DAB ON A LITTLE BIT

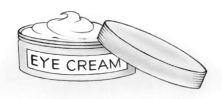

Eye Cream
Day and Night

PAMPER YOUR EYES DAILY WITH
SPECIAL CREAM FOR THIS TENDER AREA.

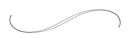

Tip#23

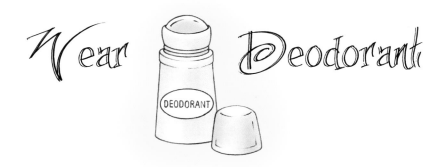

Wear Deodorant

DO WE EVEN HAVE TO GIVE
AN EXPLANATION
FOR THIS ONE?

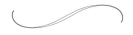

Drink Water

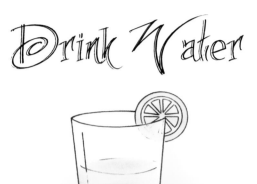

YOU HAVE HEARD IT OVER AND OVER
HYDRATE YOURSELF

Tip#25

Take Your Vitamins

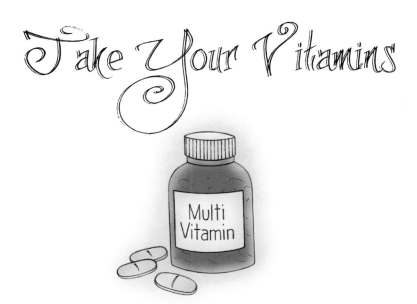

THESE LITTLE DAILY SUPPLEMENTS WILL HELP NOW
AND AS YOU AGE; THEY MAY EVEN
PREVENT SERIOUS ILLNESS

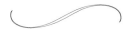

Tip #26

Eat Your

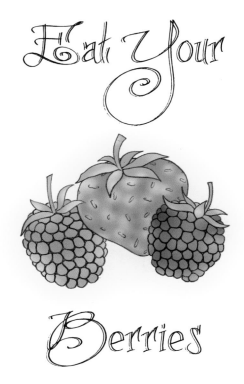

Berries

STRAWBERRIES, BLACKBERRIES, RASPBERRIES, ETC.
THESE LITTLE GUYS ARE FULL OF
FABULOUS ANTIOXIDANTS

Tip #27

Cut Preservatives

and Sodium

JUST BECAUSE PRESERVATIVES ARE
THE MAIN INGREDIENT IN ALL
THOSE SALTY SNACKS
DOESN'T MEAN THEY WILL
PRESERVE YOUR SKIN

35

Tip #28

Don't Smoke

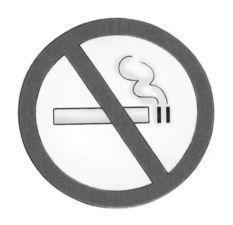

PREMATURE WRINKLES
ARE SO NOT CHIC

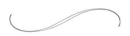

Tip#29

Spritz on Perfume

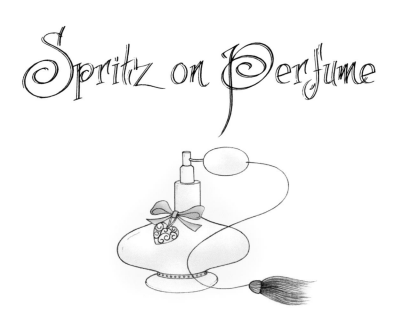

FIND A SIGNATURE SCENT TO BE REMEMBERED BY AND CARRY IT WITH YOU TO FRESHEN UP

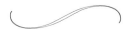

Make-up
Quick Change

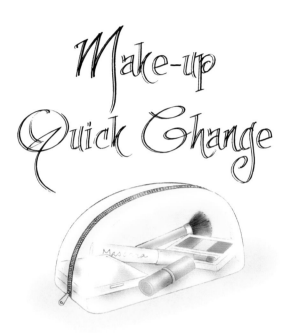

SEASONALLY CHANGE YOUR MAKE-UP
TO GO WITH WINTER AND SUMMER SKIN TONES

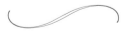

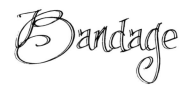

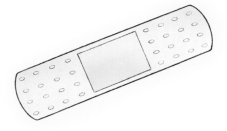

KEEP 'EM HANDY; SO USEFUL FOR
PAPER CUTS, BLISTERS, A QUICK FALLING HEM,
OR TO COVER UNMENTIONABLES IN A COOL BREEZE

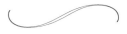

Drink Red Wine

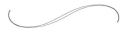

WHY NOT LOOK CHIC
WHILE ENJOYING A GLASS OF ANTIOXIDANTS

Wear a Luxurious Robe

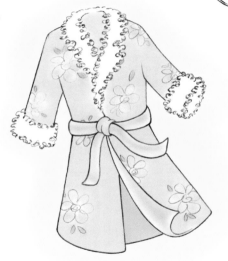

SLIP INTO A PLUSH ROBE
AND FEEL LIKE A MOVIE STAR

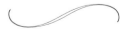

Tip #34

Send Flowers to Yourself

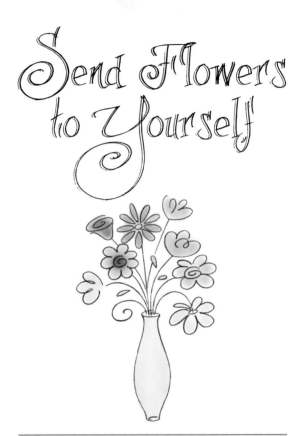

THERE IS NOTHING LIKE THE SMELL OF FRESH FLOWERS; IT LIGHTENS YOUR MOOD IN SECONDS

Tip #35

Drink Tea

THIS WARM DRINK IS FULL OF ANTIOXIDANTS
A FEW SIPS A DAY MAY KEEP THOSE BAD AILMENTS AWAY

Tip#36

5 Minute

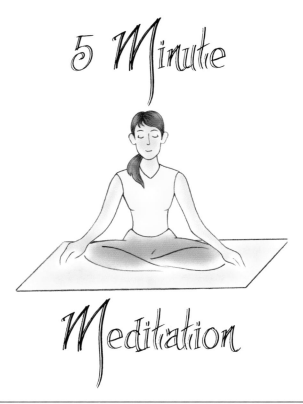

Meditation

THIS SIMPLE ACT EVERY DAY WILL INVOKE
A DEEPER STATE OF RELAXATION AND AWARENESS

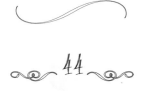

Tip #37

Walk It Out

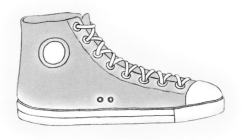

RELIEVE STRESS, TONE UP AND SIMPLY
FEEL GOOD WITH A BRISK WALK

Tip #38

Go to the Gym

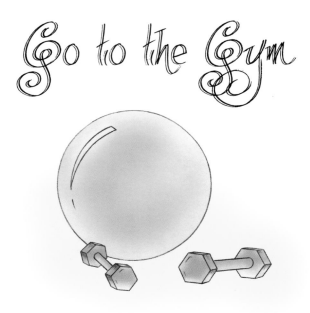

HOW MANY TIMES DO YOU HAVE TO BE TOLD
THE GYM IS GOOD FOR YOU?

Tip #39

Indulge in

Sweets

WHO DOESN'T NEED A LITTLE SOMETHING DELECTABLE TO LIGHTEN THE MOOD?

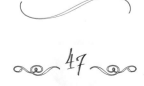

Take a Bath

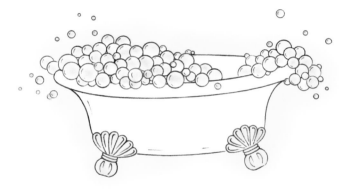

LUXURIATE IN A WARM BUBBLE BATH
STEP OUT FEELING LIKE A MILLION BUCKS

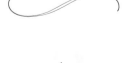

Tip#41

Love

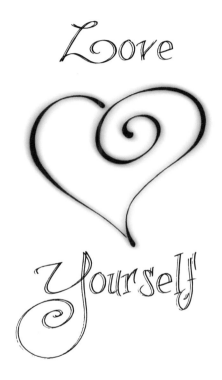

Yourself

I MEAN REALLY, IF YOU DON'T,
WHO WILL?

49

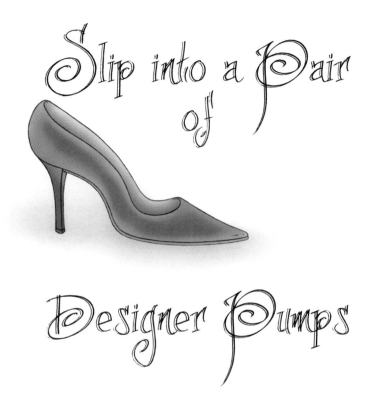

Tip #42

Slip into a Pair of

Designer Pumps

OH HOW YUMMY

EVERY GIRL SHOULD OWN AT LEAST ONE PAIR, RIGHT?

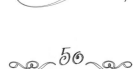

Tip #43

Accessorize

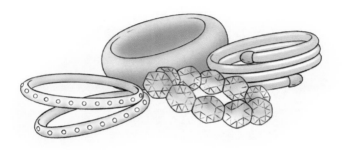

BANGLES, NECKLACES, FAUX BAUBLES CAN INSTANTLY CHANGE THE TONE OF YOUR LOOK

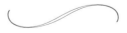

Tip #44

Invest in a Tailor

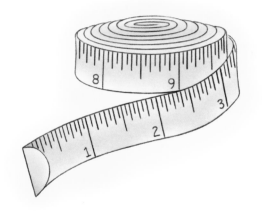

A GOOD TAILOR CAN BE A SAVIOR AND YOUR ULTIMATE RESOURCE FOR LOOKING FABULOUS IN ALL YOUR CLOTHES

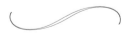

Tip#45

Carry an

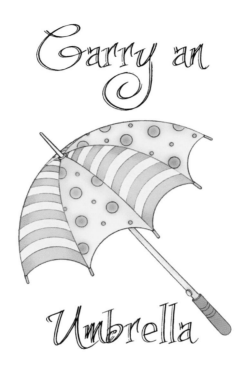

Umbrella

YOU NEVER KNOW WHEN RAIN
WILL TRICKLE DOWN, OR THE SUN WILL SHINE
A LITTLE TOO BRIGHT

Tip #46

Statement Watch

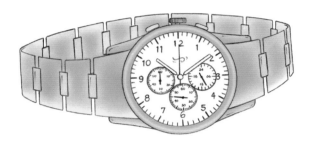

BUY A SUPER CHIC BOLD
MEN'S STYLE WATCH

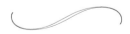

Tip #47

Watch a Classic

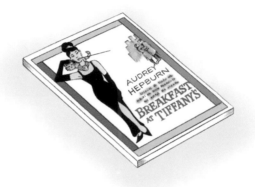

BREAKFAST AT TIFFANY'S IS WONDERFUL FOR INSPIRATION

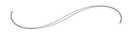

Tip #48

Buy a Classic

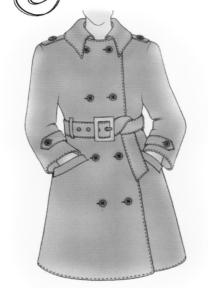

Trench Coat

THIS PIECE IN A WARDROBE
IS LIKE A FASHION ICON!

Tip#49

Visualize Your Life

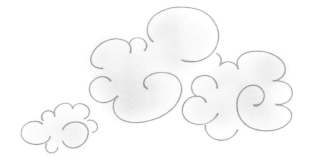

ALL THE WORLD'S POSSIBILITIES
WILL INSTANTLY COME INTO EXISTENCE

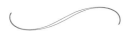

Tip #50

Hear the Music

WHO SAID OUR LIVES SHOULDN'T
EMULATE A MOVIE SOUNDTRACK

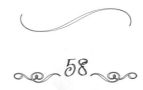

Tip#51

Find Your Muse

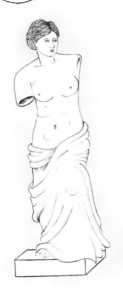

SHE MAY BE YOUR INSPIRATION
FOR YOUR NEXT GREAT ACCOMPLISHMENT

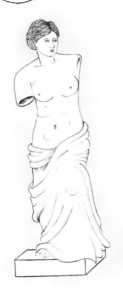

Tip #52

Be Yourself

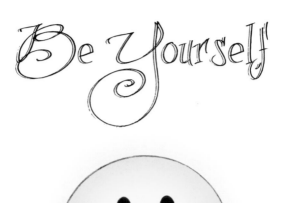

No one likes an imitation of the real thing

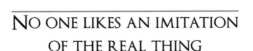

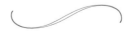

Tip #53

Find the

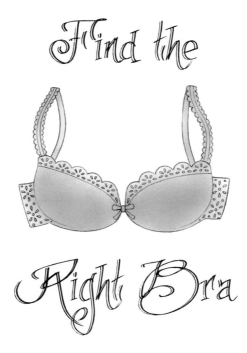

Right Bra

GET MEASURED BY A PROFESSIONAL
HOW YOU LOOK ON THE OUTSIDE
STARTS UNDERNEATH IT ALL

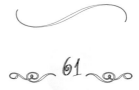

Tip#54

Splurge on a

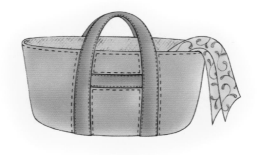

Timeless Tote

WHY DO YOU THINK YOUR GRANDMOTHER'S
CLASSIC DESIGNER BAG IS THE ENVY
OF YOUR FRIENDS?

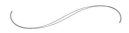

Tip #55

Buy a Jersey

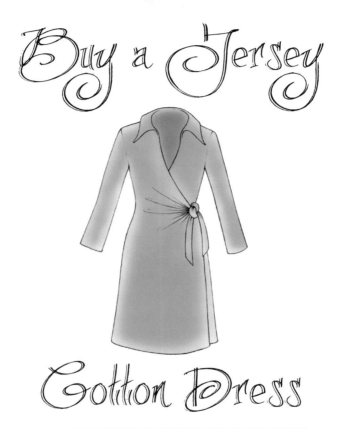

Cotton Dress

ONE OF THE MOST VERSATILE ITEMS
AND IS SUPER PERFECT FOR TRAVEL
WON'T WRINKLE!

Re-invent Your Wardrobe

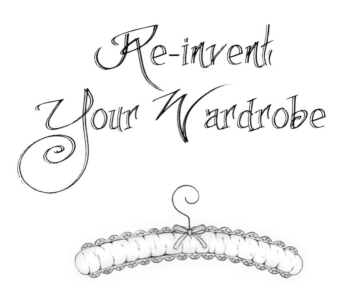

WHY CAN'T THAT OLD SUIT BE SEPARATED TAILORED AND WORKED INTO 2 DIFFERENT LOOKS?

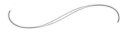

Tip#57

Beauty Rest

A LITTLE EXTRA SLEEP IS LIKE AN OVERNIGHT FACE LIFT

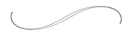

Closet Clean Up

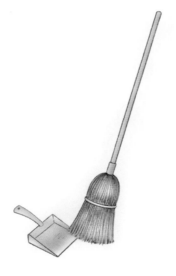

CLEARING OUT THE OLD
MAKES ROOM FOR THE NEW
AND WE GLAM GIRLS LIKE NEW

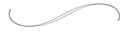

Tip #59

Stylist-On-Call

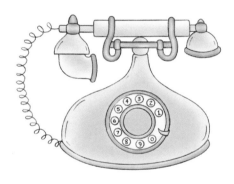

ALWAYS HAVE YOUR STYLIST
A PHONE CALL AWAY

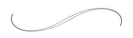

Tip#60

Signature Look

× 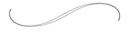 _____

_____

**FIND YOUR STYLE
AND OWN YOUR LOOK**

Take Vitamin E

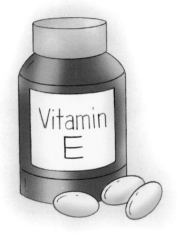

THIS WONDERFUL LITTLE VITAMIN
WILL WORK WONDERS
FOR YOUR SKIN, HAIR AND NAILS

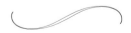

Tip#62

Exfoliate and

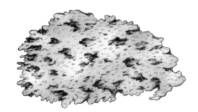

Moisturize

DON'T YOU WANT SUPER SILKY
BABY SOFT SKIN?

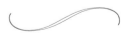

Indulge in a Facial

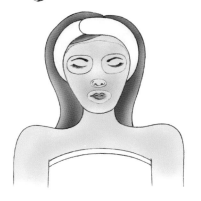

OHHH THE GLAMOROUS FEELING OF A
STEAMY FACIAL WILL MAKE ANY GIRL
FEEL LIKE A PRINCESS

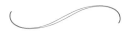

Massage Once a Month

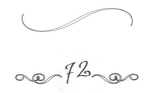

LOOSEN UP MUSCLES AND RELAX
YOU DESERVE IT

Fresh Cut Flowers

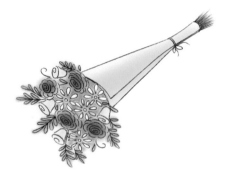

KEEP THEM AROUND YOUR HOME
FOR A FRESH SMELL AND PRETTY POPS OF COLOR

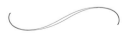

Tip #66

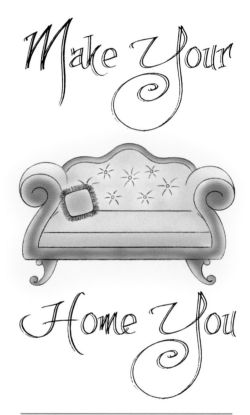

Make Your Home You

YOUR HOME SHOULD HAVE
LITTLE ACCENTS THAT REFLECT A PART OF YOU

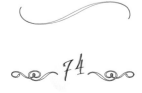

Tip #67

Stock Up On White Tanks

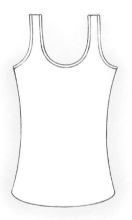

THEY CAN BE WORN WITH
ALMOST ANYTHING DRESSED-UP OR DRESSED DOWN
AND STILL LOOK CHIC

Tip#68

Wear a

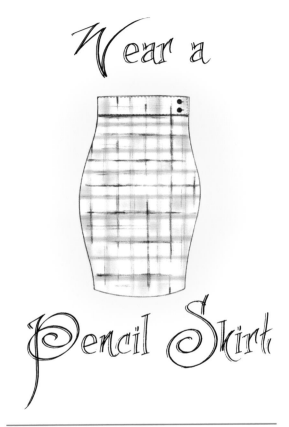

Pencil Skirt

It is an Ultra Flattering skirt
that totally hugs a woman's hourglass shape

Dress for a Red Carpet

EVEN IF YOU'RE HOME ALONE
ON A FRIDAY NIGHT, IT'S ALWAYS FUN
TO DRESS RED CARPET STYLE, SO DO IT UP!

Make Life a Special Occasion

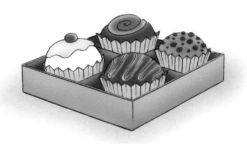

EVERY DAY SHOULD BE TREATED
LIKE A SPECIAL OCCASION, SO GO AHEAD,
TREAT YOURSELF!

Tip#71

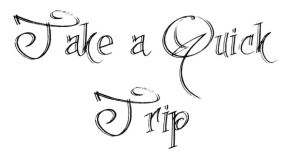

Take a Quick Trip

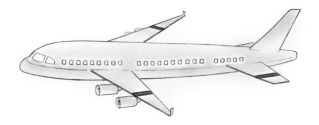

IT ALWAYS MAKES YOU FEEL LUXURIOUS
PLAN A LAST MINUTE GETAWAY

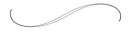

79

Tip #72

Smile

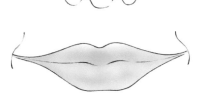

As soon as you let a little smirk out you instantly feel lighter than air

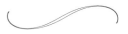

Tip#73

Mints

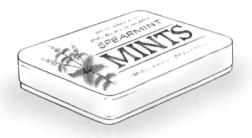

FRESH BREATH IS ALWAYS A "DO"

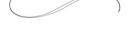

Look Polished

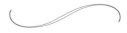

LOOKING PUT TOGETHER
ALL THE TIME
PUTS YOU ONE STEP AHEAD
OF THE CROWD

Tip#75

Reapply

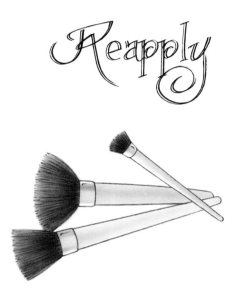

WHY DO YOU THINK STARLETS
ALWAYS LOOK SO GOOD...
IT IS ALL ABOUT REAPPLYING
LIP GLOSS THROUGH THE DAY

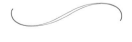

Write a Note

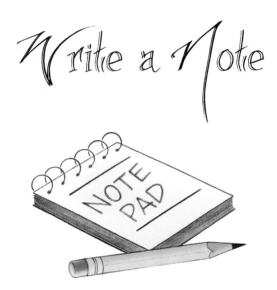

A HANDWRITTEN NOTE IS A HAPPY GREETING
IN THIS NEW DIGITAL WORLD

Tip#77

Coddle Yourself with

Egyptian Cotton

YOU SPEND MANY HOURS IN BED
IT'S ONLY RIGHT TO HAVE THE BEST SHEETS

85

Don't Lose Your Cool

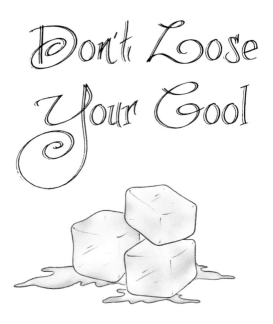

COUNT TO 10
BREATH AND DO IT AGAIN
IF YOU HAVE TO

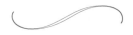

Tip #79

Keep a Journal

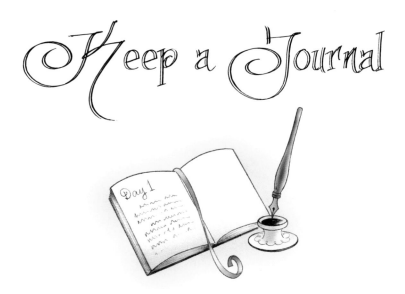

KEEP ALL YOUR HEARTFELT THOUGHTS
ON PAPER; THIS IS WHERE MEMORIES ARE STORED
AND DREAMS ARE CREATED

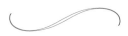

Tip#80

Vision Boards

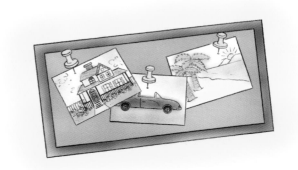

CREATE A BOARD TO DISPLAY CLIPS
OF YOUR DREAM DESTINATIONS,
HOMES, CARS AND LIFE
AND IT WILL BECOME A REALITY!

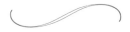

88

Tip#81

Give A little

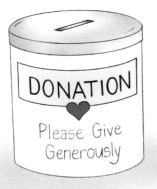

FIND A CHARITY CLOSE TO YOUR HEART
AND YOU WILL FIND A NEW OUTLOOK ON LIFE

Tip #82

Set a Beauty Routine

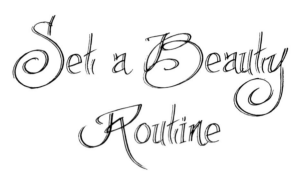

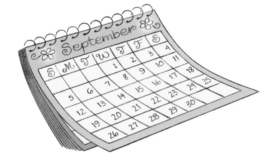

TO TAKE CARE OF YOUR SKIN

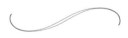

Tip#83

No Pantyhose

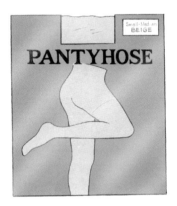

LET'S LEAVE THESE IN THE PAST
OPAQUE TIGHTS ARE THE ONLY EXCEPTION LADIES!

Tip#84

Dark Wash Denim

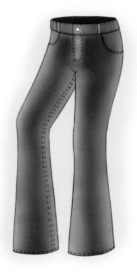

FADED COLORS ONLY MAKE YOU LOOK LARGER
STICK TO THE DARK SIDE

Tip #85

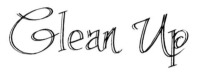

Clean Up

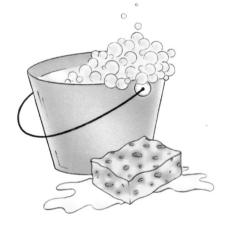

KEEP YOUR LIVING, WORK AND
TRAVEL SPACE (HOTEL ROOMS) READY FOR
VISITORS AT ANY TIME

Tip #86

Learn How to Listen

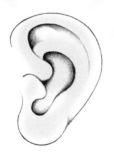

THERE'S A REASON WHY YOU HAVE
TWO EARS AND ONE MOUTH

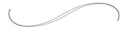

Think Hollywood Glamour

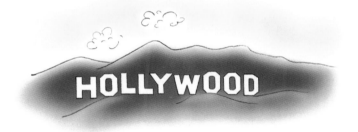

IT'S SOPHISTICATED AND GIVES
YOU AN AIR OF CONFIDENCE!

Tip#88

Change Your Mind

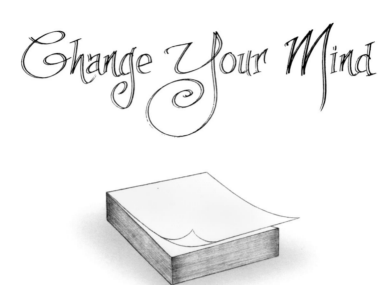

Leave little notes of motivational thoughts in places you will see them constantly

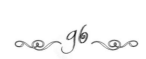

Add Animal Print

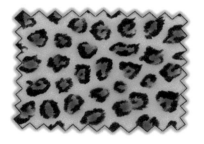

A CARPET, A HEADBAND, A PIECE OF NOTE PAPER
BRING OUT THE WILD SIDE BY
ADDING THIS PRINT TO YOUR LIFE

Tip#90

Safety Pin It

FOR QUICK FIXES, BRA STRAP MALFUNCTIONS
OR EVEN TO POP A LOCK
KEEP A SAFETY PIN IN YOUR WALLET

Brand Yourself

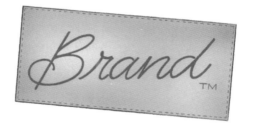

CREAT A BRAND OF YOUR OWN
WHO SAYS YOU CAN'T BE KNOWN
FOR THE STAR YOU ARE

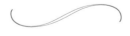

Secret Fix Double Stick Tape

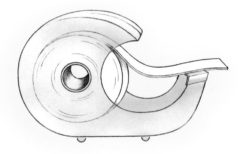

FIX PLUNGING NECKLINES, FIX BRA STRAPS
AND SHORTEN A HEM IN A PINCH

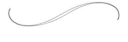

Emergency 100

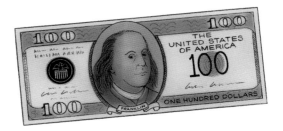

TUCK A $100 DOLLAR BILL IN A SECRET WALLET
POCKET FOR AN EMERGENCY...
AND THAT DOESN'T MEAN A
SHOPPING EMERGENCY!

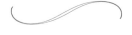

Tip #94

Invest Wisely

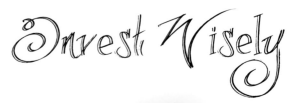

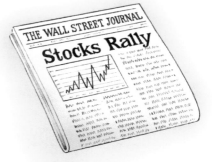

HAVE A LITTLE NEST EGG SAVINGS SOCKED AWAY FOR A RAINY DAY

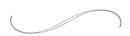

Travel Upgrades

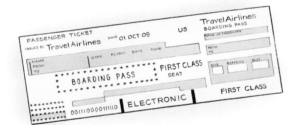

PAMPER YOURSELF. ASK FOR AN
UPGRADE TO FIRST CLASS, A CONVERTIBLE CAR
ON VACATION, OR A ROOM WITH A VIEW

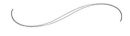

Tip #96

A Dab of Petroleum Jelly

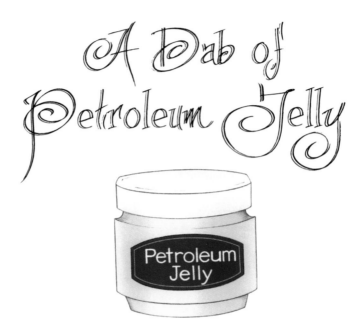

PAT SOME ON AROUND THE EYES
AND YOU WILL HAVE NO WORRIES LATER
ON WHEN YOUR ARE WRINKLE FREE

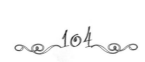

Tip#97

Throw a
Theme Party

THERE IS NOTHING LIKE AN OLD SCHOOL 50'S BASH
OR VINTAGE FLAPPER AND GENTS FETE

105

Flaunt a Beach

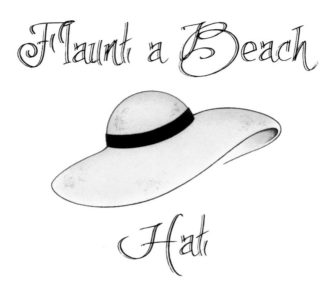

Hat

WHAT'S MORE GLAMOROUS OR SOPHISTICATED
THAN HIDING MYSTERIOUSLY BEHIND
A WIDE BRIM HAT?

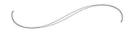

Tip #99

Stretch in the

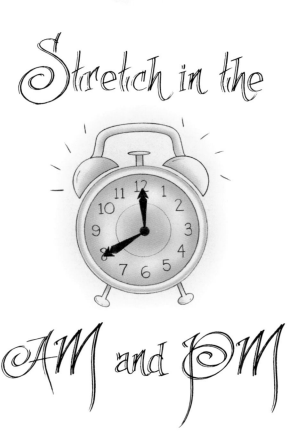

AM and PM

STAY LIMBER AND GET YOUR BLOOD FLOWING
EXCELLENT FOR CIRCULATION

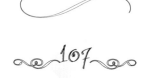

Feng Shui

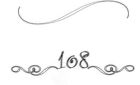

Your Home

CREATE BALANCE AND CALM IN THE SPACE
YOU SPEND MOST OF YOUR TIME

Tip#101

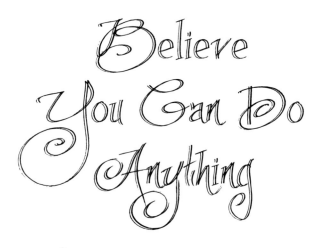

Believe
You Can Do
Anything

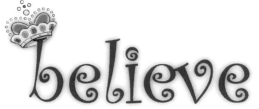

believe

REMEMBER WHAT YOU THINK YOU BECOME!

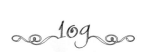

Made in the USA